DELBERT GOODWIN

Calisthenics For Beginners

Build Lean Muscles And Everlasting Strength

Contents

Introduction

What is Calisthenics?

I imagine if you're reading this book then you either have some knowledge or no knowledge of what calisthenics is. Truth be told if you've ever participated in any organized sports team then you have most likely performed some aspect of calisthenics. If you've never participated in any kind of organized sport, then I am very excited that you have chosen to purchase a copy of this book. I want to warn everyone now, however, that this will not be a comprehensive book on the full scope of calisthenics. This will be just enough to sate your curiosity and set you on the correct path to building a lean and strong body that you can be proud of.

I have to admit when it comes to calisthenics I am 100% biased. I have always preferred calisthenics over weight lifting. I am not discrediting
weight lifting or any of the benefits that come with lifting weights, however, from my experience calisthenics produces the best long term results. Why do I say that you might ask? It's because the strength and the physique that you build for your body last a lot longer, and you have a greater sense of true strength. I have personally met guys who can bench press 350 lbs and yet they can't do 100 push-ups non stop. I've seen guys that can curl 175+ lbs and yet they can't perform 20 pull-ups consecutively. To me, that's just embarrassing. Being able to do body weight exercises and do them in large quantities is the sign of

true strength.

Benefits of Calisthenics

Don't get me wrong, even though I say all of that against weight lifting. I still lift weights myself. Especially when it comes to doing lower body workouts. I tend to favor weight lifting for my lower body workouts because I easily get bored with doing high repetitions of the various leg workouts that I know. That's enough of my rant on calisthenics versus weight lifting. Let's get to the heart of the matter. Just what is Calisthenics?

Calisthenics is quite simply any workout that a person can perform with little to no equipment. Said person is literally using their own body weight to provide resistance to whatever exercise that is being performed. You will need a pull bar for pull ups and dip bars for performing dips. The thing that I love most about calisthenics are the benefits; which are: 1.) affordable and convenient (doesn't require a gym membership), 2.) easy to modify the workouts according to the level of skill/body control that you possess currently, 3.) utilizes compound exercises-meaning that you work multiple muscle groups with just one exercise, 4.) It requires a lot of movement which allows one to burn a lot of calories in a short amount of time. Which allows people to develop really lean and defined muscle groups. Calisthenics also improve flexibility, coordination, balance, and muscle endurance.

Top 5 Upper Body Workouts

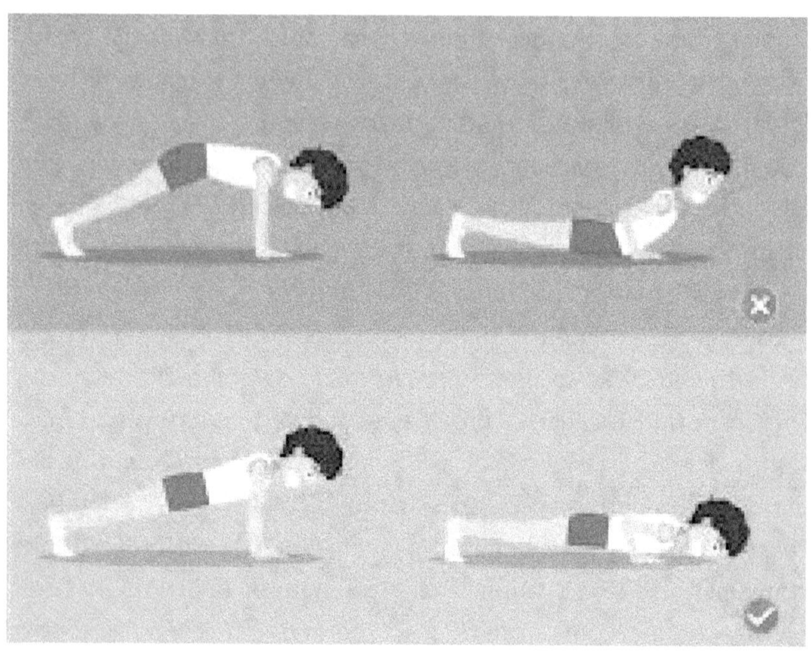

Push-up

The push-up is one of the foundational exercises that anyone will perform when exercising. There are over 10 different variations of the push-up and for the most part they target different areas of the upper body. For the purposes of this book I won't be going into detail of all the various forms of the various exercises,but I do want you to know that each exercise has more than one variation of the exercise. It's a big part of the reason why I love calisthenics so much as well. You have so many different ways that you can mix up your routine, and that you should mix up your routine. It's called muscle confusion. After doing the same exercise for about a week or two your body will get accustomed to the exercise and you will plateau. Plateau simply means that your body no longer finds the exercise to be challenging. At this point you have a couple of different options. You can either increase the repetitions or change up the variation of the exercise. There is no right or wrong answer in this case. It's all up to the individual and how hard you want to push your limits.

To perform a standard push-up you simply lay with your stomach flat on the ground with your legs extended down and the tips of your toes touching the ground. Then you position your arms into an L position at your shoulder length. Next, you just push up off the ground while attempting to keep your back straight,and then lower your body back down to the ground. If your back flexes inward or outward then you can't count that repetition as a successful repetition.

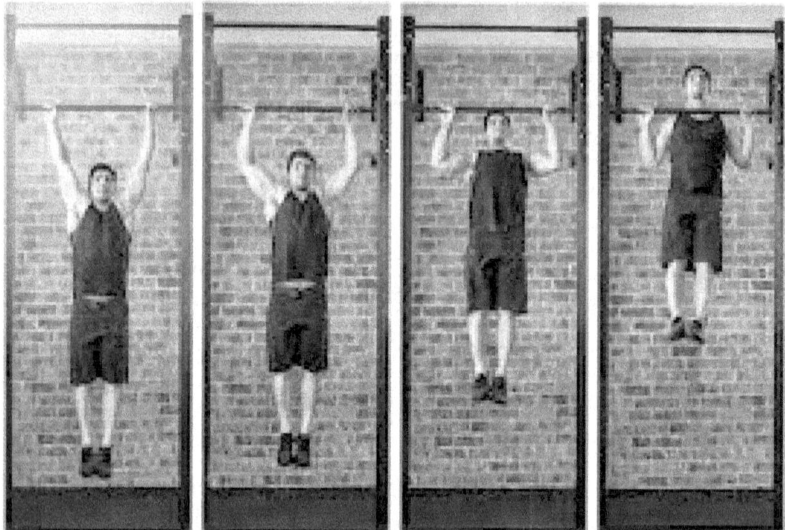

Pull up

The pull-up is another foundational exercise in terms of performing calisthenics. I remember going through the initial training to be a paratrooper for the U.S. military. One of the first things that they require you to do is to perform a single pull up and hold it for several seconds. The reason for that is because each soldier needs to have the bare minimum strength in order to pull the lines in order to guide the parachute to the ground by going either against the wind or with the wind. It all depends on where you want to land. The pull-up is in my opinion the third hardest body weight exercise known to man, the hardest being the muscle-up followed by the burpee(which won't be covered in this book). The reason that the pull-up is so difficult is because you are literally defying gravity by pulling the entirety of your bodyweight up towards the bar. How much you weigh has a direct impact on the degree of difficulty in performing a pull-up. From my experience, the more a person weighs (300 lbs+) the fewer pull-ups that he/she will be able to perform.

In order to perform a proper pull-up you start by hanging from the bar. Next, you want to position your hands shoulder width apart on the bar. Finally, you want to straighten and stiffen your legs while pulling your body up towards the bar. Be mindful not to kip (swing your legs in order to gain momentum upward). While some may count that as a successful pull-up if you kip with it, I personally do not count that as a successful pull-up.

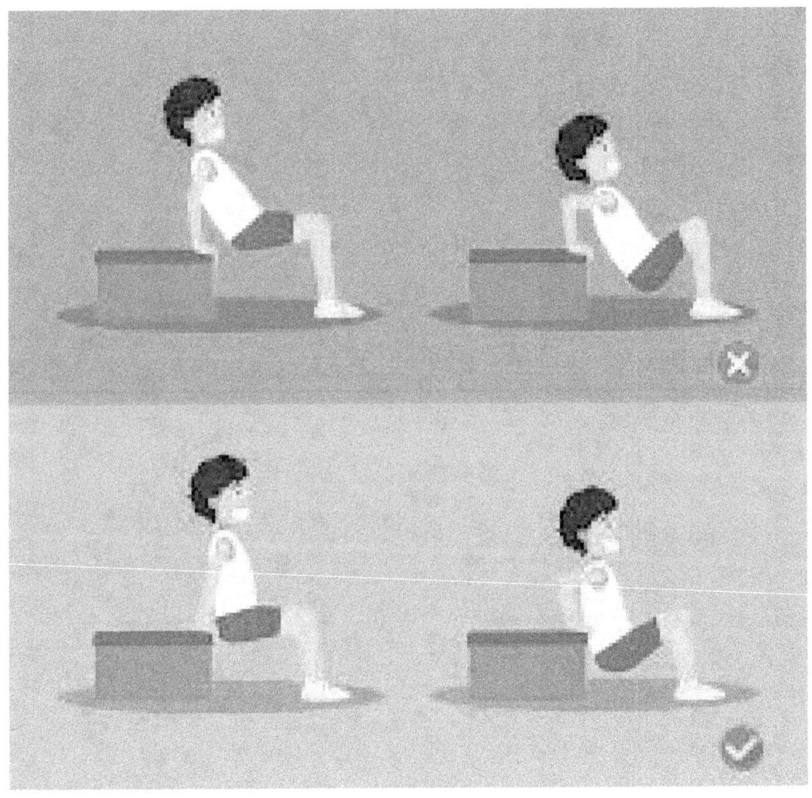

Dips

Performing a dip is almost like performing a push-up in terms of the compound muscle groups that are involved in performing a dip. In order to successfully perform a dip you should position yourself in between the dip bars. Next, you want to grab hold of the dip bar and then push up lifting your body weight onto the bars. At this point you should curl your feet (depending on how high/low your dip bars position you above the ground). Next, you lower your body down in between the dip bars and then push your body back up above the dip bars. You also want to be careful not to swing your body around too much. The more control you have over your body, the greater the benefits to your muscles are as you perform this exercise.

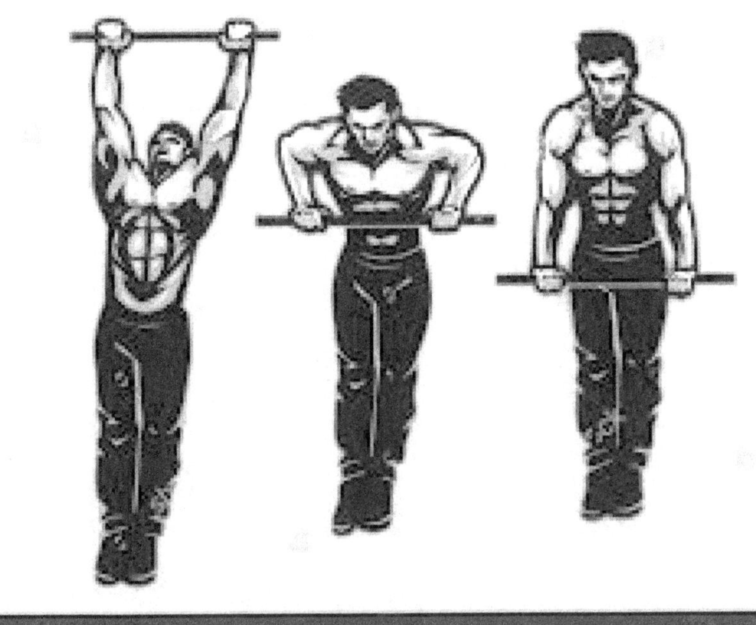

Muscle Up

The muscle up is the single most difficult free weight exercise known to man. It requires you to position yourself as though you were going to do a pull-up. As a matter of fact, in order to perform a muscle up you have to have great upper body strength and coordination. Becoming pretty great at the number of repetitions of pull-ups will definitely help build up the strength that you require in order to perform a muscle up. As I stated earlier, in order to perform a muscle up you want to start out as though you were going to do a pull up.

Now the mechanics behind doing a muscle up sounds easy,however, it is by no means easy for those with inadequate upper body strength.

I encourage you to look up videos on youtube in order to get a visual of how a muscle up is performed. I encourage this method in order to hopefully prevent you from injuring yourself when attempting to perform a muscle up. As you pull yourself up on the pull-up bar you
want to pull your entire body up and over the pull-up bar in one motion. Don't try to slowly pull your body up and over as that will just place more strain on your body. It has to be in one quick and flawless motion.

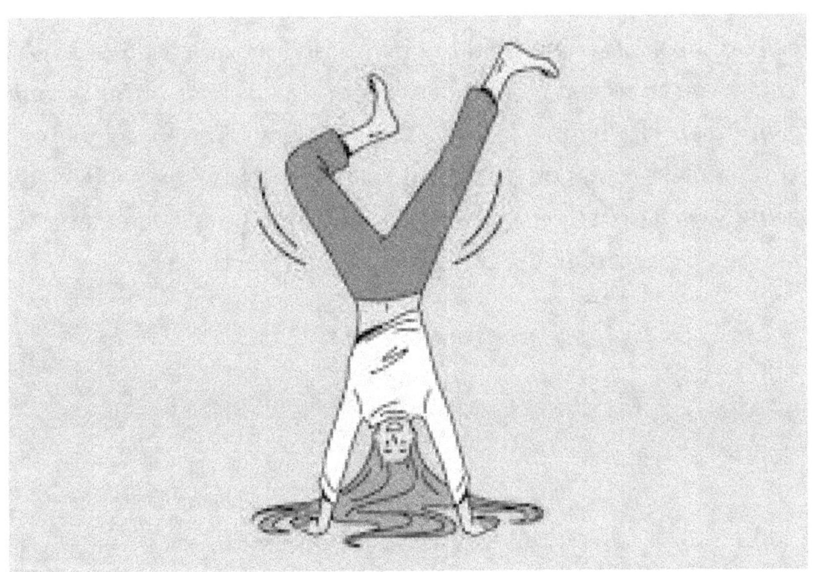

Handstand

To be honest, I still can't perform a handstand to this day. It's not that it's impossible. It's just not an exercise that I have ever really placed much importance in. However, I do understand the benefits of being able to perform a handstand. It's all about balance and muscle coordination. The best of the best when it comes to calisthenics have amazing body control and balance. Perhaps after writing this book I

will put more effort into being able to perform a handstand.

In order to build your strength so that you can perform a handstand like the top calisthenics athletes you can start by using a wall. The easiest way to begin is to face the wall and walk your legs up the wall. Try to hold the handstand for at least 5 seconds. You'll want to repeat this for five sets of five seconds or for as long as you can last before falling. Once you have gotten competent with doing handstands facing the wall, try performing handstands facing away from the wall. Repeat the repetitions the same as before. Five sets of five seconds handstands, if not longer.

Top 5 Core Workouts

13

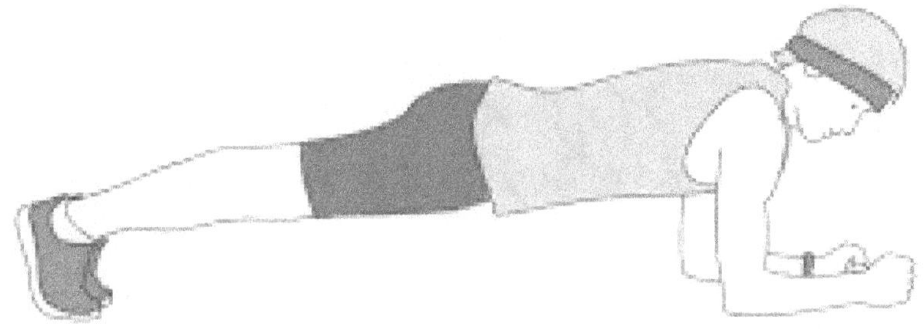

Plank

I personally don't like the plank exercise but it is a very good exercise for your core. It builds strength and balance at the same time. The plank is all about "time under tension". The longer you hold the plank the better results you will get. In order to perform a proper plank you should lay in the prone position (belly to the ground) and then raise your body onto your forearms. As you're holding your bodyweight, you also want to squeeze your core- this is where the "time under tension" comes into play. I for one didn't get into the plank exercise until after I joined the Georgia Army National Guard. This exercise is implemented in one of the core exercises that is standard when performing core exercises.

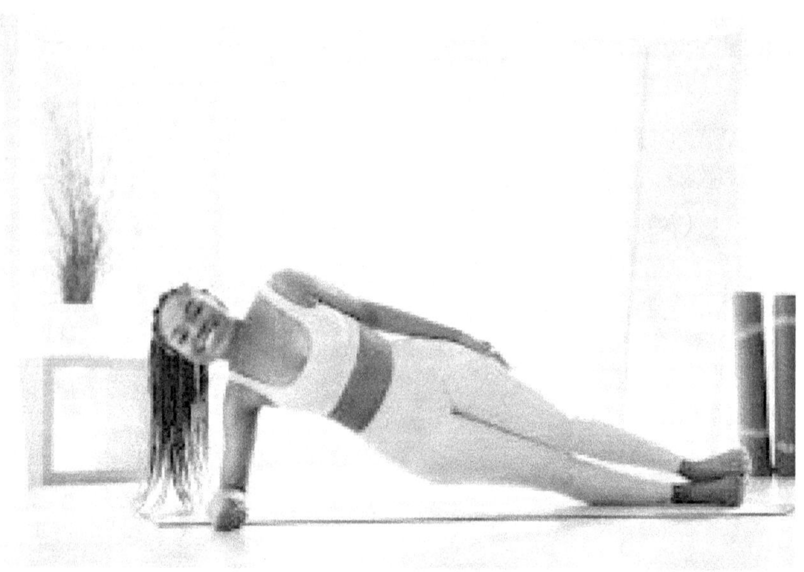

Side Plank

The side plank is a variation of the plank exercise. The difference between the plank and the side plank is literally the fact that you are turned to the side. With this exercise you want to start by laying on either your right or left side. After you have determined which side you want to workout, place the same elbow on the ground in an L shape. Your arm should be perpendicular to your body. Push off with your desired arm and keep your knees and feet together. Your feet should be stacked on top of one another. This is just like the plank position in the fact that it is "time under tension based".

SIT-UPS
Classic Sit-Ups

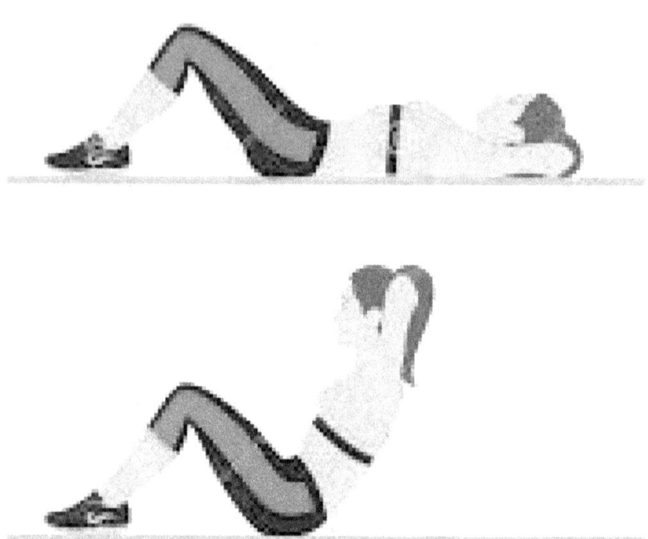

Sit-up

The sit up is the most recognized and the most basic core exercise known to mankind. It is performed by laying in the supine position (back on the ground) first. Then you want to bend your knees into a loose "L shape". Now the next part is about preference. You can either interlock your fingers behind your head and bring your body up to your knees, or you can place your hands across your chest and then lift your body up towards your knees. There are many other variations in which you can perform a sit up as well,but we'll just stick with the basics for the purposes of this book.

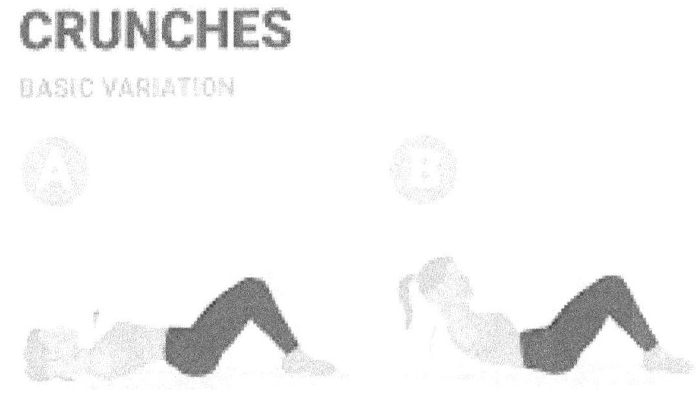

Crunch

I love the crunch. It's less stress on your back and it's easy to do. Plus you get killer definition in your top two of six abs by performing this exercise. You want to start out by laying on your back and curl your legs into your body to form a loose "L" shape again (just like the sit-up). Raise your chin towards your core and tighten your core at the same time. Feel that burn yet? That's the feeling of weakness leaving the body!

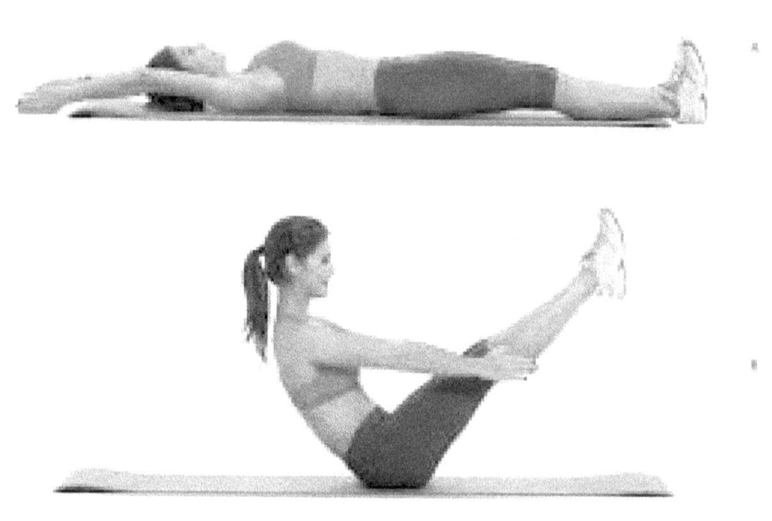

V-up

The V-up is another exercise that I came to know of after joining the military. Before that I had never heard or seen anyone perform a v-up. This is a core exercise that I also love to do. It works the entire core.

You top four and the lower two abs all get some stress placed on them during this particular exercise. To perform this exercise you need to start out in the neutral position, which is lying supine on the floor. After that you want to pull your upper body towards your knees, while at the same time pulling your legs towards your chest- without bending your knees. You want to keep your legs locked out and form a "V" with both your lower body and upper body (your arms should be extended out towards your feet).

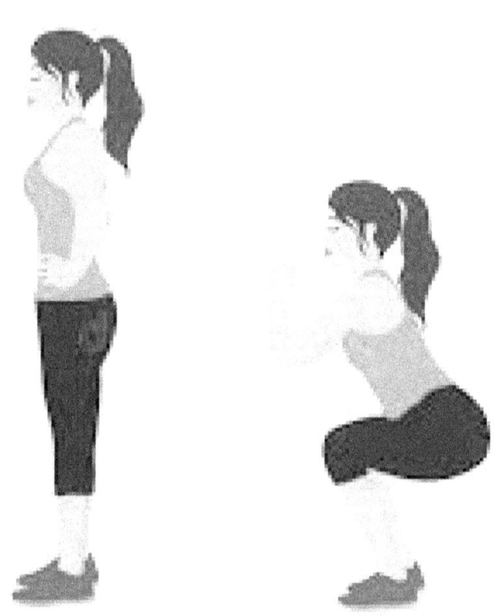

Squat

The Squat! If you've ever played an organized sport then you should be very acquainted with the squat. If not, then you're in for a treat. Both men and women love this exercise, albeit for different reasons. While both men and women love the exercise to improve their leg strength, women love the exercise because it tones up their buttocks. So for those ladies that want to get a "butt lift"; this is the exercise for you! To perform the perfect squat you want to imagine yourself sitting down in a chair. Spread your feet shoulder width apart and then squat down into a "seated position". Word to the wise, it's not a full squat unless you put your "buttocks to the ground". That means that it's a deep squat.

And trust me, you will feel it on your way back up.

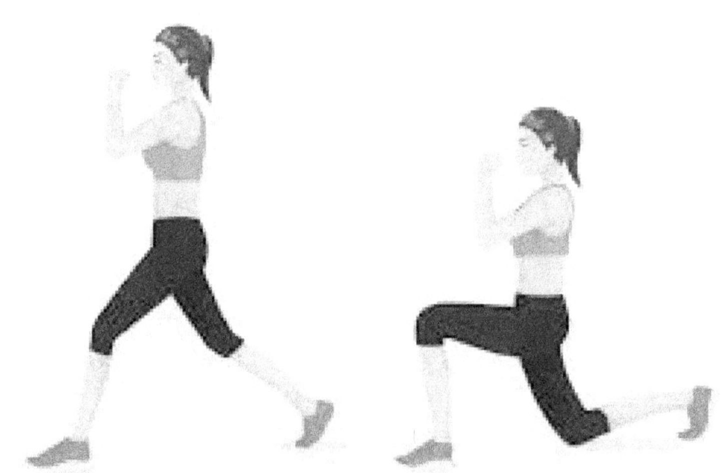

Lunge

The lung is also a staple of leg workouts. Especially when discussing calisthenics. The lunge is a very fun and versatile workout. To perform a lunge you want to stand with your back straight and chest out. Then you want to step forward or backward into the lunge. Make sure to get pretty deep with the lunge so that you can engage your quad when you push back up out of the lunge. The step forward should be bigger than the step backward. Or at least that's how I always perform my lunges,but you can take just as big a step backward as you do going forward for the rear lunge.

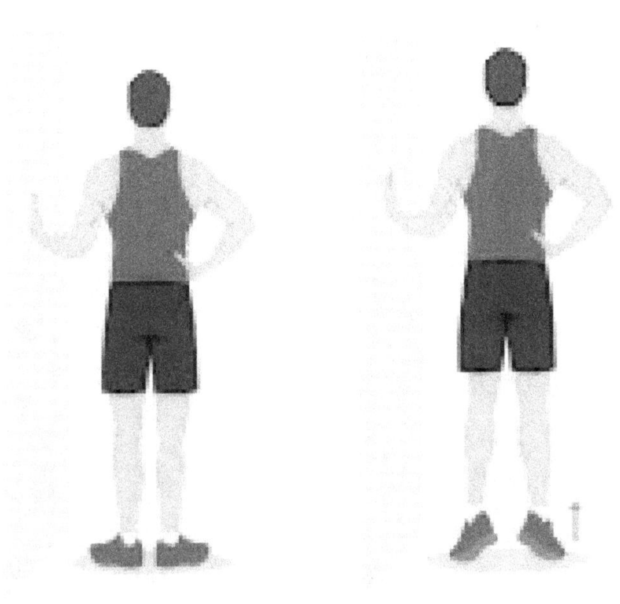

Calf Raise

Women will probably favor this workout more so than men. Typically what I have seen from men is that they incorporate the calf raise into the squat exercise instead of just doing calf raises as a solo workout. It can be done either way. To perform a proper calf raise you can simply stand against a wall or just stand upright wherever you are. You want to then raise the heel of your feet off the ground while keeping the front part of your feet on the ground. You should feel a strain in your calf muscles if done properly. You can get really sexy looking legs with this workout!

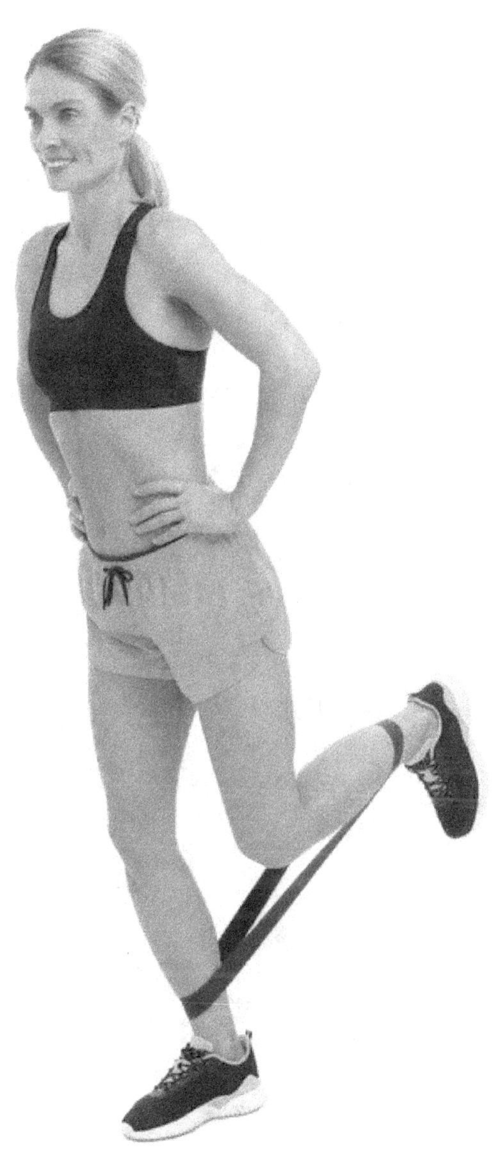

Hamstring Curl

The hamstring curl is the bane of my existence! I have naturally small legs and it seems as though no matter what I do, my legs just won't grow in mass. It's a hereditary thing. My father's legs are the exact same way. We both have some really strong legs,but you wouldn't be able to tell from just looking at them. Now this is probably the one exercise where I would encourage you to get a set of resistance bands and incorporate them into this workout. Doing hamstring curls without any kind of resistance won't yield you very great results. To perform a hamstring curl you want to either stand up straight or lay down on your stomach. The goal is to curl your leg into your body. In other words while laying on your stomach, you want to bring your leg backwards up to your buttocks. You would do the same thing if you elected to stand and perform this exercise.

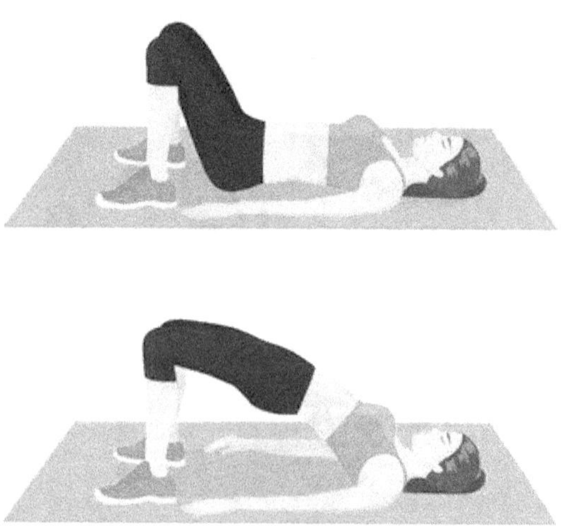

Bridge

Speaking frankly, the bridge exercise is not one of my favorite exercises.

However, it has nothing to do with the degree of difficulty, it's just that I simply don't like it. It's probably one of the few calisthenic exercises that I find to be boring. Why then did I decide to include this exercise in the book? Because this book is to expose beginners to the wonderful world of calisthenics and while I may find it to be boring that doesn't mean that everyone else does. There are some pretty amazing benefits to doing bridges. Such as: it's great for the glutes, hamstrings, and for strengthening your back and core muscles. To perform bridges correctly you want to start off as though you're going to perform a sit up. You want to have your legs in an "L" shape and then lift your buttocks into the air and hold. This is also another one of those "time under tension" exercises.

Variations of the Basics

As promised earlier, I won't go into detail on the variations of all the basic calisthenic exercises, however, I will disclose some of the variations so that once you begin to plateau you already have knowledge of how to create that muscle confusion discussed earlier.

Push-up Variations:
Decline push-up
Incline push-up
Clap push-up
Spiderman push-up One
hand push-up diamond
push-up handstand
push-up

Core Variations:
Russian twist
Mountain Climbers
Scissor Kicks
Bicycle Crunch
Flutter Kicks
Toe Touches
Reverse crunch

Lower Body Variations:

Jumping squat

Jumping lunges

Pistol squat

Split squat

Side lunges

Box jumps

High Knees

Training Program

Sets, Repetitions, Hold Times

You can get very creative with how you complete calisthenic workouts. You can do 2 - 4 sets of 5, 10,15, 20, 25, etc. of whichever exercise you choose. For those "time under tension" workouts such as the plank, side plank, and the bridge; you want to hold those for anywhere from 30 seconds, 1 minute, 1 minute and 30 seconds, and/or 2 minutes. If you're really feeling frisky then try holding it for as long as you possibly can. "Time under tension" or hold times aren't just limited to the three exercises that I just mentioned. You can complete it with any exercise. The key to it is your level of comfort. How far do you want to push your limits? "Time under tension" doesn't just mean holding the exercise for a certain amount of time. It also means going slow with the exercise. It ties into a concept known as negatives. Completing a negative is when you're going back to the neutral position of any exercise and you take your time getting back to the neutral position. That's combining "time under tension" and "negatives". Talk about a slow burn! But you will see massive results in your strength. "Negatives" and "time under tension" is the main ingredient to building that everlasting strength that was mentioned on the cover of this book.

You don't really want to do any more than 4 sets of any exercise. The reason why I recommend no more than four sets is so that you mentally don't get burned out. Calisthenics is just as much mental as it is physical. You have to pump yourself up as you progress through the sets, repetitions, and hold times.

31

Conclusion

32

As you have probably come to understand by now, the world of calisthenics is very versatile and multidimensional. It most certainly is not a group of workouts that you can put into a "proverbial box". People have gotten really creative and flexible with the workouts that they have come up with so far. Keep in mind that I have only scratched the surface of what all you can do with calisthenics. There are many more variations of all these basic exercises that I have covered with you. I encourage you to do your own research and discover just how " deep the rabbit hole goes".

Thanks for taking the time to read my book. I know that it wasn't the most comprehensive guide to calisthenics but it is my hope that it has sparked a desire and a willingness to dive deeper into calisthenics and all that it has to offer. You can consider calisthenics as the "natural/organic"
way to build muscle as opposed to weight lifting. If you don't mind. I would really love it if you would leave a review for this book. I enjoyed writing it and I hope you enjoyed reading it as much as I did writing it!

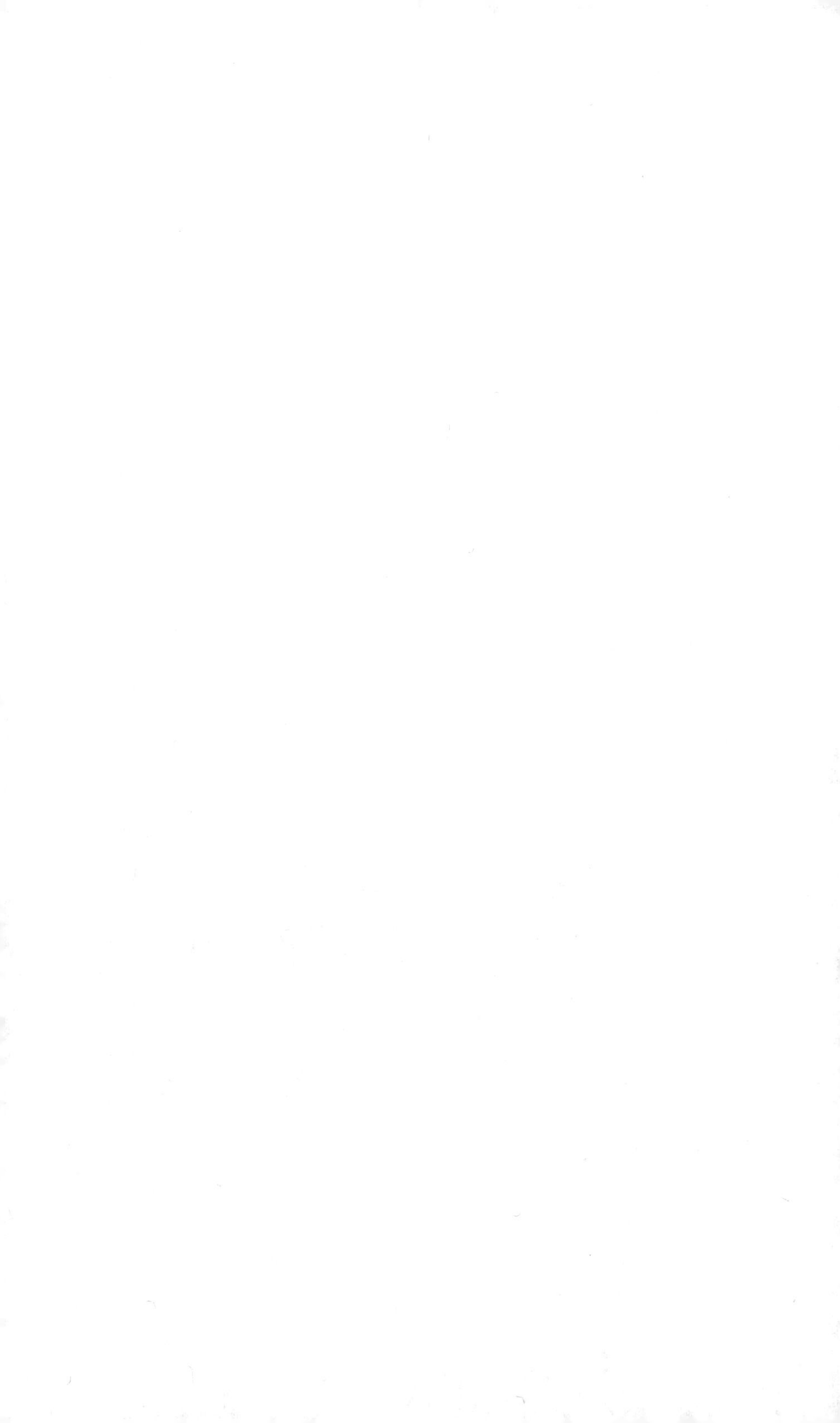